CONQUERING HIGH BLOOD PRESSURE

A Holistic Approach to Hypertension Management

ADOOH MARCEL

DEDICATION

This book is dedicated to God almighty and my entire family for their unwavering support, boundless encouragement, and profound love they have showered upon me throughout my life and in the course of writing this book. They are the beating heart of my existence, and I want the world to know just how profoundly I appreciate their presence in my journey. And I pray that the almighty God bless them all.

Contents

INTRODUCTION

Hypertension, often referred to as the silent killer, is a formidable adversary that silently creeps into the lives of millions around the world. This relentless dragon, with its ability to wreak havoc on our health, often goes unnoticed until it's too late. In this battle against hypertension, it's crucial to arm ourselves with knowledge and awareness, and to stand ready to face this formidable opponent head-on.

Hypertension, or high blood pressure, is a condition in which the force of blood against the walls of the arteries is consistently too high. While it may not manifest with obvious symptoms, its impact on our overall health is profound. Left uncontrolled, hypertension can lead to severe health complications, including heart disease, stroke, kidney problems, and more.

This silent dragon doesn't discriminate; it can affect anyone, regardless of age, gender, or background. It's not just a concern for the elderly but a growing issue among young adults and even children, thanks to lifestyle factors and genetic predisposition.

Our journey to facing the hypertension dragon begins with understanding its origins, recognizing its warning signs, and adopting strategies to control it. We must equip ourselves with the knowledge of healthier eating habits, regular physical activity, and stress management, as these are the tools that will empower us to fend off this menacing beast.

Throughout this journey, we'll explore the causes and risk factors of hypertension, learn about its devastating consequences, and discover practical steps to maintain optimal blood pressure and overall well-being. Together, we'll arm ourselves with the knowledge and tools necessary to confront the hypertension dragon, ensuring that we live our lives to the fullest without being held captive by this silent threat. It's time to embark on this critical battle and emerge victorious against hypertension.

CHAPTER ONE
DEFINING HYPERTENSION

Hypertension, commonly known as high blood pressure, is a medical condition characterized by elevated and sustained blood pressure in the arteries. Blood pressure is the force of blood pushing against the walls of the arteries as the heart pumps it throughout the body. When this pressure is consistently higher than normal, it is classified as hypertension.

Blood pressure is typically measured in millimeters of mercury (mm Hg) and is expressed as two numbers, such as 120/80 mm Hg. These numbers represent:

1. **Systolic Pressure:** The top number, which represents the pressure in the arteries when the heart beats and pumps blood into the circulatory system.
2. **Diastolic Pressure:** The bottom number, which represents the pressure in the arteries when the heart is at rest between beats.

Normal blood pressure is usually considered to be around 120/80 mm Hg. However, the optimal range can vary depending on individual factors, and healthcare providers may use slightly different criteria.

Hypertension is typically categorized into several stages:

1. **Normal Blood Pressure:** Less than 120/80 mm Hg.
2. **Elevated Blood Pressure:** A systolic pressure between 120-129 mm Hg and a diastolic pressure less than 80 mm Hg.
3. **Hypertension Stage 1:** A systolic pressure between 130-139 mm Hg or a diastolic pressure between 80-89 mm Hg.
4. **Hypertension Stage 2:** A systolic pressure of 140 mm Hg or higher or a diastolic pressure of 90 mm Hg or higher.

5. **Hypertensive Crisis:** A severe and potentially life-threatening condition where blood pressure is 180 mm Hg or higher for the systolic pressure and/or 120 mm Hg or higher for the diastolic pressure. Immediate medical attention is necessary in this case.

Hypertension is a significant risk factor for various health problems, including heart disease, stroke, kidney disease, and damage to blood vessels. It is often called the "silent killer" because it can develop over time without noticeable symptoms. Regular blood pressure monitoring and appropriate management are essential to prevent and control hypertension and its associated health risks. Treatment may involve lifestyle modifications, such as dietary changes and exercise, and, in some cases, medication prescribed by a healthcare professional.

TYPES AND CAUSES OF HIGH BLOOD PRESSURE

High blood pressure, or hypertension, can be categorized into two main types based on its causes: primary (essential) hypertension and secondary hypertension. Both types can have multiple contributing factors, and sometimes the exact cause may not be clear. Here's an overview of these types and their causes:

1. **Primary (Essential) Hypertension:** is the most common form of high blood pressure, accounting for the majority of cases. The exact cause of primary hypertension is often unknown, but it's believed to be the result of a combination of genetic, lifestyle, and environmental factors.

   Common contributing factors to primary hypertension include:
   - **Genetics:** A family history of hypertension can increase the risk.
   - **Age:** As people get older, the risk of developing hypertension increases.

- **Diet:** A diet high in salt (sodium) and low in potassium, as well as excessive alcohol consumption, can raise blood pressure.
- **Obesity:** Being overweight or obese puts extra stress on the cardiovascular system.
- **Physical Inactivity:** Lack of regular exercise can contribute to hypertension.
- **Stress:** Chronic stress can play a role in elevating blood pressure.
- **Smoking:** Tobacco use can temporarily raise blood pressure and damage blood vessels.
- **Insulin Resistance and Metabolic Syndrome:** Conditions related to insulin resistance, obesity, and abnormal lipid profiles can contribute to hypertension.

2. **Secondary Hypertension:** is less common than primary hypertension and is typically a result of an underlying medical condition or medication.

Identifiable causes of secondary hypertension may include:

- **Kidney Problems:** Kidney diseases or disorders, such as renal artery stenosis, glomerulonephritis, or polycystic kidney disease, can lead to hypertension.
- **Hormonal Issues:** Conditions like primary aldosteronism, Cushing's syndrome, or thyroid disorders can affect blood pressure.
- **Medications:** Some drugs, such as nonsteroidal anti-inflammatory drugs (NSAIDs), birth control pills, decongestants, and certain prescription medications, can lead to elevated blood pressure.
- **Obstructive Sleep Apnea:** This sleep disorder can be associated with hypertension.
- **Endocrine Tumors:** Rare tumors can produce hormones that lead to high blood pressure.

- **Pregnancy-Induced Hypertension:** Conditions like preeclampsia can cause high blood pressure during pregnancy.
- **Illegal Drugs:** The use of drugs like cocaine and amphetamines can lead to hypertension.
- **Dietary Supplements:** Some dietary supplements, such as ephedra and licorice, may cause an increase in blood pressure.
- **Chronic Alcohol Abuse:** Long-term excessive alcohol consumption can lead to hypertension.

It's crucial to identify and address the underlying cause of secondary hypertension, as treating the root condition can often lead to blood pressure control. If you suspect you have high blood pressure or have been diagnosed with it, consult with a healthcare professional for a thorough evaluation, appropriate testing, and personalized treatment and lifestyle recommendations. Controlling high blood pressure is essential for reducing the risk of serious health complications.

THE HIDDEN DANGERS IN HIGH BLOOD PRESSURE

High blood pressure, or hypertension, is often called the "silent killer" because it can develop without obvious symptoms but still pose significant dangers to your health. Here are some of the hidden dangers associated with high blood pressure:

1. **Heart Disease:** High blood pressure can damage the arteries and heart over time. This can lead to conditions like coronary artery disease, heart attacks, and congestive heart failure.
2. **Stroke:** Hypertension is a leading cause of strokes. Elevated blood pressure can damage the blood vessels in the brain, increasing the risk of both ischemic (clot-related) and hemorrhagic (bleeding) strokes.
3. **Kidney Damage:** The kidneys rely on healthy blood vessels to filter waste from the blood. High blood pressure can damage the blood vessels in the kidneys, leading to kidney disease and, in severe cases, kidney failure.

4. **Eye Problems:** Hypertension can damage the blood vessels in the eyes, leading to vision problems or even blindness. It may contribute to conditions such as retinopathy.
5. **Aneurysms:** Weak spots in blood vessels can develop, forming aneurysms. When these aneurysms rupture, they can be life-threatening, depending on their location.
6. **Peripheral Artery Disease:** High blood pressure can damage the blood vessels in the extremities, reducing blood flow to the legs and arms. This can result in pain, poor wound healing, and, in severe cases, gangrene.
7. **Cognitive Decline:** Some studies suggest a link between hypertension and cognitive decline, including an increased risk of Alzheimer's disease and other forms of dementia.
8. **Metabolic Syndrome:** Hypertension is often associated with other metabolic risk factors, including obesity, high cholesterol, and insulin resistance. These factors collectively increase the risk of heart disease and diabetes.
9. **Sexual Dysfunction:** High blood pressure can contribute to erectile dysfunction in men, affecting sexual health and quality of life.
10. **Preeclampsia:** Pregnant women with uncontrolled hypertension can develop a condition called preeclampsia, which can be life-threatening for both the mother and baby.
11. **Reduced Life Expectancy:** Uncontrolled hypertension is a significant contributor to premature death. It shortens life expectancy and increases the risk of severe health complications.
12. **Emotional and Psychological Impact:** Living with high blood pressure can be emotionally and psychologically taxing. It can lead to anxiety and stress, affecting overall well-being.

To avoid these hidden dangers, it's crucial to monitor your blood pressure regularly and work with a healthcare professional to manage and control hypertension. Lifestyle modifications, such as a heart-healthy diet, regular exercise, stress reduction, and medication, if necessary, can help maintain healthy blood pressure levels and reduce the risk of these hidden health complications. Early detection and intervention are key to preventing the serious consequences of high blood pressure.

Conquering High Blood Pressure

THE IMPORTANCE OF TAKING ACTION ON HIGH BLOOD PRESSURE

Taking action on high blood pressure is of paramount importance because uncontrolled hypertension can have serious and potentially life-threatening consequences. Here are some key reasons why it is vital to address high blood pressure promptly:

1. **Reducing the Risk of Cardiovascular Disease:** High blood pressure is a leading risk factor for heart disease, including conditions like heart attacks, angina, and heart failure. By managing blood pressure, you significantly reduce the risk of these cardiovascular events.
2. **Stroke Prevention:** Hypertension is a major risk factor for strokes, including ischemic (caused by blood clots) and hemorrhagic (caused by bleeding) strokes. Proper blood pressure control can lower the likelihood of a stroke.
3. **Kidney Health:** High blood pressure can damage the blood vessels in the kidneys, leading to kidney disease and eventually kidney failure. Controlling blood pressure helps protect kidney function.
4. **Vision Protection:** Hypertension can cause damage to the blood vessels in the eyes, leading to vision problems and even blindness. Managing blood pressure can help safeguard your vision.
5. **Reducing the Risk of Aneurysms:** Weakened blood vessels due to high blood pressure can lead to the development of aneurysms (ballooning of blood vessels). If these burst, it can be life-threatening. Blood pressure management reduces this risk.
6. **Improving Overall Quality of Life:** High blood pressure, when left untreated, can lead to fatigue, shortness of breath, chest pain, and other symptoms that reduce your quality of life. Proper management can help you feel better and more energetic.
7. **Preventing Cognitive Decline:** Some studies suggest a link between hypertension and cognitive decline, including an increased risk of Alzheimer's disease. Maintaining healthy blood pressure may help protect cognitive function.
8. **Enhancing Longevity:** Addressing high blood pressure can significantly increase your life expectancy. Uncontrolled hypertension is a significant contributor to premature death.

9. **Lowering Healthcare Costs:** Managing blood pressure can lead to reduced healthcare expenses in the long run. Treating hypertension is generally less costly than managing the consequences of uncontrolled high blood pressure.

10. **Personal Well-Being:** High blood pressure can be a source of anxiety and stress. Taking action to control it not only benefits your physical health but can also improve your mental and emotional well-being.

Taking action on high blood pressure typically involves lifestyle changes, such as a heart-healthy diet, regular exercise, weight management, stress reduction, and limiting alcohol and sodium intake. Medications may also be prescribed by a healthcare provider to help lower blood pressure.

It's essential to monitor your blood pressure regularly and work closely with your healthcare provider to develop a personalized plan for managing high blood pressure. By taking action, you can protect your health, prevent life-threatening complications, and improve your overall well-being.

CHAPTER TWO
UNDERSTANDING HIGH BLOOD PRESSURE READINGS

Understanding high blood pressure readings is essential for managing this condition effectively. Blood pressure is typically expressed as two numbers, such as 120/80 mm Hg, and each number has its significance:

1. **Systolic Pressure (Top Number):** This represents the pressure in your arteries when your heart beats and pumps blood into the circulatory system. It's the higher of the two numbers.
2. **Diastolic Pressure (Bottom Number):** This represents the pressure in your arteries when your heart is at rest between beats, or in other words, the pressure in your arteries when the heart is not actively pumping blood. It's the lower of the two numbers.

UNDERSTANDING YOUR BLOOD PRESSURE READING:

- **Normal Blood Pressure:** A normal blood pressure reading is typically around 120/80 mm Hg. In this case, 120 is the systolic pressure, and 80 is the diastolic pressure. It indicates that your blood pressure is within a healthy range.
- **Elevated Blood Pressure:** An elevated blood pressure reading falls between 120-129 mm Hg for systolic and less than 80 mm Hg for diastolic. It suggests that your blood pressure is higher than normal, and you should take steps to prevent it from rising further.
- **Hypertension Stage 1:** If your blood pressure is between 130-139 mm Hg for systolic or 80-89 mm Hg for diastolic, you have stage 1 hypertension. At this stage, lifestyle changes are often recommended, and medication may be considered, depending on your individual risk factors and health.
- **Hypertension Stage 2:** A reading of 140 mm Hg or higher for systolic, or 90 mm Hg or higher for diastolic, indicates stage 2 hypertension. It is a more severe form of high blood pressure and typically requires medication along with lifestyle modifications.

- **Hypertensive Crisis:** If your blood pressure is 180 mm Hg or higher for systolic or 120 mm Hg or higher for diastolic, you are in a hypertensive crisis. This is a medical emergency, and you should seek immediate medical attention. It may be associated with symptoms like severe headache, shortness of breath, chest pain, or confusion.

It's important to note that blood pressure guidelines may vary slightly between healthcare organizations, so consult with your healthcare provider to determine your specific target range. They will consider your individual health factors, such as age, sex, and any underlying medical conditions, to determine the best approach for managing your blood pressure.

Regular monitoring of your blood pressure and working with a healthcare professional to develop a personalized plan for managing high blood pressure are essential steps in maintaining your cardiovascular health and preventing related complications.

THE ROLE OF HYPERTENSION IN HEALTH

Hypertension, or high blood pressure, plays a significant role in health, both positive and negative. Understanding this role is essential for managing the condition effectively and maintaining overall well-being. Here's an overview of the various aspects of the role of hypertension in health:

NEGATIVE ROLE OF HYPERTENSION:

1. **Cardiovascular Disease:** High blood pressure is a major risk factor for heart disease, including conditions such as coronary artery disease, heart attacks, and congestive heart failure. It can lead to the narrowing and hardening of arteries (atherosclerosis), making it more challenging for the heart to pump blood effectively.
2. **Stroke:** Hypertension is a leading cause of strokes, both ischemic (clot-related) and hemorrhagic (bleeding) strokes. Elevated blood

pressure can damage the blood vessels in the brain, increasing the risk of these potentially life-threatening events.

3. **Kidney Damage:** Uncontrolled hypertension can damage the blood vessels in the kidneys, leading to chronic kidney disease and, in severe cases, kidney failure. The kidneys play a crucial role in filtering waste from the blood.

4. **Eye Problems:** High blood pressure can damage the blood vessels in the eyes, potentially leading to vision problems or even blindness. Conditions like hypertensive retinopathy can result from prolonged elevated blood pressure.

5. **Aneurysms:** Weak spots in blood vessels can develop into aneurysms. When these aneurysms rupture, they can be life-threatening, depending on their location. Hypertension contributes to the risk of aneurysm formation.

6. **Peripheral Artery Disease:** Hypertension can damage blood vessels in the extremities, reducing blood flow to the legs and arms. This can lead to pain, impaired wound healing, and, in severe cases, gangrene.

7. **Metabolic Syndrome:** Hypertension is often associated with other metabolic risk factors, including obesity, high cholesterol, and insulin resistance. These factors collectively increase the risk of heart disease and diabetes.

8. **Cognitive Decline:** Some studies suggest a link between hypertension and cognitive decline, including an increased risk of Alzheimer's disease and other forms of dementia.

9. **Reduced Life Expectancy:** Uncontrolled hypertension is a significant contributor to premature death. It shortens life expectancy and increases the risk of severe health complications.

POSITIVE ROLE OF HYPERTENSION:

While hypertension is primarily considered detrimental to health, it also plays a somewhat protective role in certain situations. For example, during acute stress or sudden blood loss, a temporary increase in blood pressure can help redirect blood flow to vital organs and ensure oxygen delivery. This is part of the body's "fight or flight" response.

Conquering High Blood Pressure

However, chronic, long-term hypertension is where the negative health implications become more prominent. It's crucial to address and manage hypertension effectively through lifestyle modifications and, when necessary, medication prescribed by a healthcare provider. Early detection and intervention are key to preventing the serious consequences of high blood pressure and maintaining overall health.

CHAPTER THREE
THE POWER OF DIET AND NUTRITION IN MANAGING HIGH BLOOD PRESSURE

Diet and nutrition play a powerful role in managing and preventing high blood pressure (hypertension). Making the right food choices and adopting a heart-healthy diet can have a significant impact on blood pressure levels. Here are some key principles for harnessing the power of diet and nutrition to control high blood pressure:

1. **Reduce Sodium (Salt) Intake:**
   - Excessive sodium consumption can lead to high blood pressure because it causes the body to retain water, which increases blood volume and pressure.
   - Limit processed and fast foods, as they are often high in hidden sodium.
   - Opt for fresh, whole foods, and use herbs and spices to season your meals instead of salt.
2. **Increase Potassium Intake:**
   - Potassium helps counterbalance the effects of sodium in the body and relax blood vessel walls.
   - Foods rich in potassium include bananas, oranges, potatoes, spinach, and avocados.
3. **Adopt the DASH Diet:**
   - The Dietary Approaches to Stop Hypertension (DASH) diet emphasizes fruits, vegetables, whole grains, lean protein, and low-fat dairy products.
   - It is rich in nutrients like potassium, calcium, magnesium, and fiber, which are beneficial for blood pressure control.
4. **Limit Saturated and Trans Fats:**
   - Saturated and trans fats can contribute to the buildup of cholesterol in the arteries, leading to higher blood pressure.
   - Reduce consumption of red meat, full-fat dairy products, and foods containing trans fats.

5. **Increase Fiber Intake:**
    - High-fiber foods, such as whole grains, fruits, and vegetables, can help lower blood pressure and improve heart health.
6. **Moderate Alcohol Consumption:**
    - Excessive alcohol intake can raise blood pressure. If you drink, do so in moderation (up to one drink per day for women and up to two drinks per day for men).
7. **Control Portion Sizes:**
    - Overeating, even of healthy foods, can lead to weight gain, which is a risk factor for high blood pressure.
    - Pay attention to portion sizes to avoid excessive calorie intake.
8. **Watch Your Caffeine Intake:**
    - While caffeine affects individuals differently, it can temporarily raise blood pressure. Monitor your response to caffeine and adjust your intake accordingly.
9. **Stay Hydrated:**
    - Dehydration can lead to an increase in blood pressure. Ensure you are adequately hydrated by drinking enough water throughout the day.
10. **Maintain a Healthy Weight:**
    - Achieving and maintaining a healthy weight can help lower blood pressure. A balanced diet and regular physical activity are key components of weight management.
11. **Consult a Healthcare Provider:**
    - For some individuals, specific dietary restrictions or recommendations may be necessary. If you have hypertension, consult with a healthcare provider or a registered dietitian for personalized dietary guidance.

Adopting a heart-healthy diet is a fundamental component of a comprehensive approach to managing high blood pressure. It is often most effective when combined with regular physical activity, stress management, and, in some cases, medication as prescribed by a healthcare provider. Making these dietary changes can not only help control hypertension but also improve overall cardiovascular health.

EXERCISING YOUR WAY TO LOWER BLOOD PRESSURE

Exercise is a powerful and effective way to lower and manage high blood pressure (hypertension). Regular physical activity can help improve your cardiovascular health, reduce the risk of heart disease, and contribute to better blood pressure control. Here's how you can exercise your way to lower blood pressure:

1. **Aerobic Exercise:**
   - Aerobic or cardiovascular exercise is especially beneficial for lowering blood pressure. It strengthens the heart, improves blood flow, and helps the body use oxygen more efficiently.
   - Examples of aerobic activities include brisk walking, jogging, running, swimming, cycling, and dancing.
2. **Frequency and Duration:**
   - Aim for at least 150 minutes of moderate-intensity aerobic exercise or 75 minutes of vigorous-intensity aerobic exercise per week. You can spread this over several days.
   - For more significant blood pressure reduction and overall health benefits, strive for 300 minutes of moderate-intensity exercise or 150 minutes of vigorous-intensity exercise per week.
3. **Strength Training:**
   - Strength or resistance training, which involves lifting weights or using resistance bands, can complement aerobic exercise by improving muscle strength and endurance.
   - Include strength training exercises at least two days a week. Work all major muscle groups, such as legs, arms, chest, back, and core.
4. **Flexibility and Balance Exercises:**
   - Activities that improve flexibility and balance, such as yoga or tai chi, can be valuable in reducing stress and enhancing overall well-being.
5. **Warm-Up and Cool-Down:**

- Before and after exercising, take the time to warm up and cool down. This helps prevent injury and gradually transitions your body in and out of exercise.

6. **Consistency Matters:**
   - Consistency in your exercise routine is key. Regular physical activity provides ongoing benefits for blood pressure control.

7. **Stay Hydrated:**
   - Drink plenty of water before, during, and after exercise to stay hydrated. Dehydration can affect blood pressure.

8. **Monitor Intensity:**
   - During aerobic exercise, aim for a moderate level of intensity where you can talk but not sing. You should feel your heart rate increase but not become excessively breathless.
   - If you opt for high-intensity exercise, make sure you're in good physical condition to do so safely.

9. **Consult Your Healthcare Provider:**
   - If you have pre-existing health conditions or concerns about starting an exercise routine, consult with your healthcare provider. They can provide personalized recommendations.

10. **Track Your Progress:**
    - Keep a record of your exercise routines and blood pressure readings. Monitoring your progress can be motivating and help you see the positive impact of exercise on your blood pressure.

Regular physical activity, in combination with a heart-healthy diet and other lifestyle modifications, can help you lower and control high blood pressure. It's important to remember that the benefits of exercise extend beyond blood pressure reduction, as it also contributes to better overall cardiovascular health, weight management, and stress reduction.

STRESS MANAGEMENT TECHNIQUES IN CONTROLLING HIGH BLOOD PRESSURE

Stress management is an essential component of controlling high blood pressure (hypertension) because stress can contribute to

Conquering High Blood Pressure

elevated blood pressure and exacerbate the condition. Here are some effective stress management techniques that can help you lower your stress levels and, in turn, better control your blood pressure:

1. **Deep Breathing and Relaxation Techniques:**
   - Deep breathing exercises, progressive muscle relaxation, and guided imagery can help calm the body's stress response. These techniques encourage relaxation and reduce tension.
2. **Mindfulness Meditation:**
   - Mindfulness meditation involves paying attention to the present moment without judgment. It can help you stay grounded and reduce stress. Regular meditation practice has been associated with lower blood pressure.
3. **Yoga:**
   - Yoga combines physical postures, deep breathing, and meditation. It can improve flexibility, reduce stress, and enhance overall well-being.
4. **Regular Exercise:**
   - Physical activity is not only beneficial for your physical health but also for managing stress. Exercise releases endorphins, which are natural mood lifters.
5. **Maintain a Healthy Lifestyle:**
   - A balanced diet, adequate sleep, and limiting alcohol and caffeine intake are crucial for managing stress. Avoid excessive consumption of these substances, as they can exacerbate stress and high blood pressure.
6. **Time Management:**
   - Effective time management can help reduce the feeling of being overwhelmed. Prioritize tasks, set realistic goals, and break them down into manageable steps.
7. **Social Support:**
   - Connecting with friends and loved ones can provide emotional support and reduce feelings of isolation. Sharing your concerns with others can be therapeutic.
8. **Limit Stressors:**
   - Identify sources of stress in your life and take steps to reduce or eliminate them. This might involve adjusting your work

schedule, decluttering your home, or setting boundaries with people or situations that cause stress.

9. **Hobbies and Leisure Activities:**
   - Engage in activities that you enjoy and that help you relax. This might include reading, gardening, art, music, or any other hobby that brings you joy.

10. **Professional Help:**
    - If you find it challenging to manage stress on your own, consider seeking support from a mental health professional, such as a therapist or counselor.

11. **Biofeedback:**
    - Biofeedback is a technique that helps you become more aware of your body's responses to stress. It can teach you how to control bodily functions, such as heart rate, and reduce stress.

12. **Positive Thinking:**
    - Replacing negative thoughts with positive ones can help you cope with stress more effectively. Practice self-compassion and challenge negative self-talk.

13. **Journaling:**
    - Keeping a journal allows you to express your feelings and gain insight into the causes of stress. It can be a therapeutic and self-reflective exercise.

14. **Limit Screen Time:**
    - Reducing excessive screen time, especially with exposure to news or social media, can help reduce stress.

15. **Relaxing Music and Nature Sounds:**
    - Listening to soothing music or sounds of nature can help calm your mind and reduce stress.

It's important to recognize that stress management is a personal journey, and what works for one person may not work for another. Experiment with different techniques to find the ones that resonate with you and effectively reduce your stress levels. The goal is to develop a routine that helps you manage stress and, in turn, supports better blood pressure control.

CHAPTER FOUR
MEDICATIONS FOR HIGH BLOOD PRESSURE

Medications for high blood pressure (hypertension) are commonly prescribed to help lower and control blood pressure levels when lifestyle modifications alone are not sufficient. There are several classes of medications available, each with its own mechanisms and potential side effects. The choice of medication or combination of medications depends on individual factors and the severity of hypertension. Here are some of the common classes of medications used to treat high blood pressure:

1. **Diuretics (Water Pills):**
   - Diuretics help the body get rid of excess sodium and water, reducing blood volume and, in turn, blood pressure.
   - Examples include thiazide diuretics (e.g., hydrochlorothiazide), loop diuretics (e.g., furosemide), and potassium-sparing diuretics (e.g., spironolactone).
2. **Beta-Blockers:**
   - Beta-blockers reduce the heart's workload by blocking the effects of adrenaline, which lowers heart rate and blood pressure.
   - Examples include metoprolol, atenolol, and propranolol.
3. **ACE Inhibitors (Angiotensin-Converting Enzyme Inhibitors):**
   - ACE inhibitors relax blood vessels and reduce blood volume by inhibiting the conversion of angiotensin I to angiotensin II, a substance that narrows blood vessels.
   - Examples include enalapril, lisinopril, and ramipril.
4. **ARBs (Angiotensin II Receptor Blockers):**
   - ARBs also relax blood vessels and lower blood pressure by blocking the action of angiotensin II.
   - Examples include losartan, valsartan, and irbesartan.
5. **Calcium Channel Blockers:**
   - These medications relax blood vessels and decrease the force of the heart's contractions, reducing blood pressure.

- Examples include amlodipine, nifedipine, and diltiazem.

6. **Alpha-Blockers:**
   - Alpha-blockers reduce nerve impulses that tighten blood vessels, which can help lower blood pressure.
   - Examples include doxazosin and prazosin.

7. **Alpha-Beta Blockers:**
   - These medications block both alpha and beta receptors, reducing heart rate and relaxing blood vessels.
   - Examples include carvedilol and labetalol.

8. **Vasodilators:**
   - Vasodilators directly relax the muscles in blood vessel walls, which leads to reduced blood pressure.
   - Examples include hydralazine and minoxidil.

9. **Central Agonists (Alpha-2 Adrenergic Agonists):**
   - These medications act on the central nervous system to reduce nerve signals that narrow blood vessels, leading to lower blood pressure.
   - Examples include clonidine and methyldopa.

10. **Direct Renin Inhibitors:**
    - These medications inhibit renin, an enzyme involved in the regulation of blood pressure.
    - Aliskiren is an example of a direct renin inhibitor.

It's important to note that the choice of medication may be influenced by individual factors such as age, gender, race, and any concurrent medical conditions. Your healthcare provider will consider these factors and tailor the treatment plan to your specific needs. Additionally, medication for high blood pressure is usually prescribed alongside lifestyle modifications, such as dietary changes, exercise, stress management, and weight control, to achieve the best results in blood pressure control. Regular monitoring and follow-up with your healthcare provider are crucial to ensure that your blood pressure is well-managed.

MONITORING YOUR PROGRESS WHEN TREATING HIGH BLOOD PRESSURE

Monitoring your progress when treating high blood pressure (hypertension) is crucial for managing the condition effectively and reducing the risk of complications. Here are important steps to help you keep track of your progress:

1. **Regular Blood Pressure Checks:**
   - Monitor your blood pressure as directed by your healthcare provider. This may involve at-home monitoring with a blood pressure monitor or visits to your healthcare provider's office.
   - Record your blood pressure readings, including the date, time, and the arm used for measurement.
2. **Follow Healthcare Provider's Recommendations:**
   - Adhere to your healthcare provider's treatment plan, which may include medication, lifestyle modifications, and any other prescribed therapies.
3. **Keep a Blood Pressure Log:**
   - Maintain a journal or digital record of your blood pressure readings. Tracking your readings over time can help identify trends and provide insight into the effectiveness of your treatment.
4. **Consistent Medication Use:**
   - If you are prescribed medication, take it as directed. Missing doses can lead to fluctuations in blood pressure.
5. **Lifestyle Modifications:**
   - Implement and maintain healthy lifestyle changes, such as dietary improvements, regular exercise, stress management, weight control, and limiting alcohol and sodium intake.
6. **Dietary Control:**
   - Monitor your diet to ensure that you are following any recommended dietary changes, such as reducing salt intake,

increasing potassium-rich foods, and maintaining a balanced diet.

7. **Exercise Routine:**
   - Keep a record of your physical activity, including the type, duration, and intensity of your workouts. Track your progress and celebrate milestones.

8. **Weight Management:**
   - If weight loss is part of your treatment plan, track your weight regularly to ensure that you are making progress.

9. **Stress Management:**
   - Use stress management techniques, such as meditation or deep breathing exercises, and note how they affect your overall stress levels and blood pressure.

10. **Medication Side Effects:**
    - Be aware of any potential side effects from your medication and report them to your healthcare provider. They may need to adjust your medication or prescribe an alternative.

11. **Follow-Up Appointments:**
    - Attend follow-up appointments with your healthcare provider as recommended. These visits are an opportunity to review your progress, make any necessary adjustments to your treatment plan, and ask questions.

12. **Maintain a Healthy Lifestyle:**
    - Continue to prioritize a heart-healthy lifestyle that promotes blood pressure control and overall well-being.

13. **Share Information:**
    - Communicate openly with your healthcare provider about your progress, any challenges you face, and any changes you have made to your treatment plan.

14. **Educate Yourself:**
    - Learn about hypertension and its management to make informed decisions and actively participate in your healthcare.

15. **Set Realistic Goals:**
    - Establish achievable goals for your blood pressure and overall health. Celebrate your successes along the way.

Conquering High Blood Pressure

Regular monitoring, coupled with consistent adherence to your treatment plan, is key to effectively managing high blood pressure. By tracking your progress and working closely with your healthcare provider, you can better control your blood pressure and reduce the risk of complications associated with hypertension.

BUILDING A SUPPORT SYSTEM FOR HIGH BLOOD PRESSURE

Building a strong support system for high blood pressure (hypertension) is vital for effectively managing the condition and maintaining your overall health and well-being. Here are steps to help you create a supportive network:

1. **Family and Friends:**
   - Inform your family and close friends about your hypertension diagnosis. Share your goals and treatment plan with them.
   - Ask for their support, whether it's encouragement to stick to a healthy diet or participating in physical activities together.
2. **Healthcare Provider:**
   - Establish a strong partnership with your healthcare provider. Regularly consult with them to discuss your treatment plan, progress, and any concerns or questions.
   - Ensure you understand your medications, including their dosages and potential side effects.
3. **Support Groups:**
   - Consider joining a local or online hypertension support group. These groups offer a platform for sharing experiences, advice, and encouragement with others facing similar challenges.
4. **Registered Dietitian:**
   - If dietary changes are part of your treatment plan, consult a registered dietitian. They can provide personalized guidance and help you create a practical meal plan.
5. **Exercise Partners:**

- Find a workout buddy or participate in group fitness classes. Exercising with others can make physical activity more enjoyable and help you stay motivated.

6. **Therapist or Counselor:**
   - A mental health professional can assist you in managing stress, anxiety, and emotional aspects related to your hypertension.

7. **Pharmacist:**
   - Develop a relationship with your pharmacist. They can offer valuable information about your medications, answer questions, and provide guidance on managing potential side effects.

8. **Online Resources:**
   - Explore credible online resources and websites dedicated to hypertension. These can provide information, tips, and community support.

9. **Education:**
   - Learn as much as you can about hypertension. Understanding the condition and its management will help you make informed decisions and take an active role in your healthcare.

10. **Spouse or Partner:**
    - If you have a spouse or partner, involve them in your hypertension management. Engage in healthy activities together, plan nutritious meals, and offer each other emotional support.

11. **Self-Help Tools:**
    - Use apps, wearable devices, and tools designed to help you monitor your blood pressure, track progress, and stay on top of your health goals.

12. **Community Resources:**
    - Explore local resources, such as community centers, fitness programs, or wellness classes, which may offer support for hypertension management.

13. **Keep Loved Ones Informed:**
    - Encourage your loved ones to learn about hypertension and its management, so they can better support you and understand your needs.

14. **Advocate for Yourself:**
    - Be an advocate for your health. Communicate your needs, concerns, and goals to your support system and healthcare providers.
15. **Regular Updates:**
    - Stay in touch with your support system regularly. Share your progress, discuss any challenges, and express your feelings and needs.

A strong support system can make a significant difference in your hypertension management journey. It can help you stay motivated, reduce stress, and improve your overall quality of life. Remember that your support system should be tailored to your unique needs and preferences, and it can evolve over time as your goals and circumstances change.

CHAPTER FIVE
SUCCESS STORIES FROM REAL WARRIORS ON HIGH BLOOD PRESSURE

Hypertension is a common condition, and many individuals have successfully managed and controlled their high blood pressure. While each person's journey is unique, here are a few success stories from people who have effectively managed their hypertension:

1. **John's Journey to a Healthier Lifestyle:**
   - John was diagnosed with high blood pressure in his late 40s. He decided to take action and began making changes to his lifestyle. He started with regular exercise, including walking and swimming. He also adopted a heart-healthy diet, reducing his salt intake and incorporating more fruits and vegetables.
   - Over time, John lost weight and noticed a significant improvement in his blood pressure readings. He continues to monitor his blood pressure, maintain his healthy habits, and enjoys an active and fulfilling life.
2. **Emily's Commitment to Stress Reduction:**
   - Emily's high-pressure job and busy lifestyle contributed to her hypertension diagnosis in her early 30s. She realized that managing her stress was crucial to controlling her blood pressure.
   - Emily started practicing mindfulness meditation and yoga, which helped her relax and reduce her stress levels. Along with medication, these practices have allowed her to keep her blood pressure within a healthy range.
3. **Daniel's Medication Management:**
   - Daniel's family has a history of hypertension, and he was diagnosed with high blood pressure in his early 40s. His healthcare provider prescribed medication to control his blood pressure.

- With regular check-ups and medication compliance, Daniel has successfully maintained his blood pressure within a healthy range. He emphasizes the importance of working closely with his healthcare provider and not hesitating to ask questions or express concerns about his treatment.

4. **Sarah's Weight Loss Journey:**
   - Sarah struggled with obesity, and her high blood pressure was a cause for concern. She decided to make a commitment to lose weight and improve her overall health.
   - Through a combination of dietary changes and regular exercise, Sarah lost a significant amount of weight over time. As a result, her blood pressure improved, and she was able to reduce her reliance on medication.

5. **George's Support System:**
   - George was diagnosed with hypertension after a routine check-up. He reached out to his family and friends for support in his journey to better health.
   - With encouragement from his loved ones, George made significant lifestyle changes. He engaged in regular physical activity, made dietary improvements, and attended support group meetings for individuals with high blood pressure. The combined support from his family and the support group helped him stay committed to managing his condition.

These success stories highlight the importance of individualized approaches to managing hypertension. Successful management often involves a combination of lifestyle changes, medication, stress reduction, and support from healthcare providers and loved ones. While each person's journey is different, these stories demonstrate that with determination, a proactive approach, and a strong support system, it is possible to effectively manage high blood pressure and lead a healthy, fulfilling life.

Conquering High Blood Pressure

OVERCOMING CHALLENGES WITH HIGH BLOOD PRESSURE

Overcoming challenges with high blood pressure (hypertension) can be a significant achievement, but it often requires determination, commitment, and a willingness to make lasting lifestyle changes. Here are some common challenges associated with hypertension and strategies to overcome them:

1. **Adherence to Medication:**
   - Challenge: Many individuals find it difficult to adhere to their prescribed medication regimen due to side effects, inconvenience, or forgetfulness.
   - Strategy: Discuss any concerns or side effects with your healthcare provider. They can adjust your medication or recommend alternatives. Use pill organizers or reminders to help you remember your doses.
2. **Healthy Eating:**
   - Challenge: Adopting a heart-healthy diet, reducing sodium intake, and maintaining portion control can be challenging, especially when dining out or in social situations.
   - Strategy: Plan your meals, cook at home more often, and choose restaurants with healthier menu options. Educate yourself on reading food labels and identifying hidden sources of sodium.
3. **Regular Exercise:**
   - Challenge: Finding the time and motivation for regular physical activity can be a struggle, especially with busy schedules.
   - Strategy: Incorporate exercise into your daily routine by scheduling it like any other appointment. Choose activities you enjoy to make it more enjoyable and sustainable. Consider joining a fitness class or finding a workout partner for motivation.
4. **Stress Management:**
   - Challenge: Reducing stress can be difficult, especially in high-pressure environments or during life changes.

- Strategy: Practice stress reduction techniques such as mindfulness meditation, deep breathing exercises, or yoga. Make time for hobbies and activities you enjoy. Consider professional counseling or therapy if needed.

5. **Weight Management:**
   - Challenge: Achieving and maintaining a healthy weight can be challenging due to factors like genetics, metabolism, and lifestyle.
   - Strategy: Set realistic weight loss goals and focus on gradual, sustainable changes. Consult with a registered dietitian or nutritionist for personalized guidance. Consider support from a weight loss group or buddy.

6. **Regular Monitoring:**
   - Challenge: Regularly checking your blood pressure can be tedious, and some people may avoid monitoring it.
   - Strategy: Establish a routine for monitoring your blood pressure, and track your progress to stay motivated. Use technology, such as blood pressure monitors and apps, to make monitoring easier.

7. **Social and Peer Pressure:**
   - Challenge: Social gatherings and peer pressure can make it challenging to stick to a heart-healthy lifestyle.
   - Strategy: Communicate your health goals to friends and family. Seek support from those who understand and respect your commitment. Practice assertiveness in social situations by making healthier choices.

8. **Resistance to Change:**
   - Challenge: Resistance to change is a common obstacle when transitioning to a healthier lifestyle.
   - Strategy: Start with small, manageable changes, and gradually build on them. Seek support and motivation from healthcare providers, support groups, or friends who have similar health goals.

9. **Financial Constraints:**
   - Challenge: Healthy food, fitness programs, and healthcare costs can strain your budget.

- Strategy: Look for affordable options, such as buying in-season produce or accessing free or low-cost exercise programs in your community. Consult with your healthcare provider about cost-effective medication options.

10. **Emotional Impact:**
    - Challenge: Dealing with the emotional and psychological impact of hypertension can be difficult.
    - Strategy: Seek emotional support from loved ones or consider professional counseling. Joining support groups for individuals with hypertension can provide a sense of community and understanding.

Overcoming challenges with high blood pressure often requires patience and persistence. It's important to remember that small, consistent steps can lead to significant improvements in your health. Seek support from healthcare professionals, friends, and family, and celebrate your achievements along the way.

MAINTAINING LONG-TERM VICTORY OVER HIGH BLOOD PRESSURE

Maintaining long-term victory over high blood pressure (hypertension) involves consistent efforts, lifestyle changes, and a commitment to ongoing self-care. Here are some key strategies to help you sustain your success in managing hypertension:

1. **Regular Monitoring:**
   - Continue to monitor your blood pressure regularly, as recommended by your healthcare provider. This allows you to track your progress and catch any changes early.
2. **Lifelong Commitment to Lifestyle Changes:**
   - Maintain the healthy lifestyle changes that have helped you control your blood pressure. This includes a heart-healthy diet, regular exercise, stress management, and weight control.
3. **Medication Adherence:**

- If you are prescribed medication, take it consistently as directed by your healthcare provider. Avoid skipping doses or stopping your medication without consulting your healthcare provider.

4. **Educate Yourself:**
   - Keep learning about hypertension, its management, and any new developments in treatment. Knowledge empowers you to make informed decisions about your health.

5. **Regular Check-Ups:**
   - Attend regular check-ups with your healthcare provider, even when your blood pressure is well-controlled. These appointments can help identify any potential issues early.

6. **Stress Management:**
   - Continue to practice stress management techniques as part of your daily routine. Stress can impact blood pressure, so managing it is crucial for long-term success.

7. **Social Support:**
   - Maintain your support system of family, friends, and healthcare professionals. Share your progress, concerns, and achievements with them.

8. **Celebrate Milestones:**
   - Recognize and celebrate your milestones and successes in managing your blood pressure. These can be important motivators for maintaining long-term victory.

9. **Flexibility and Adaptation:**
   - Be prepared to adapt to changes in your life, health, and needs. As you age, your body may have different requirements for managing hypertension.

10. **Consistency is Key:**
    - Consistency in your lifestyle, medication, and stress management efforts is essential for long-term success. Make these health-promoting habits a permanent part of your life.

11. **Learn from Challenges:**
    - If you face setbacks or challenges in managing your blood pressure, use them as opportunities for learning and growth. Reflect on what triggered the setback and make necessary adjustments.

12. **Stay Informed:**
   - Stay informed about new research and developments in hypertension management. Emerging treatments or lifestyle recommendations may offer even better strategies for controlling blood pressure.

13. **Advocate for Yourself:**
   - Be an advocate for your health. If you have questions or concerns about your treatment plan, communicate openly with your healthcare provider and actively participate in your healthcare decisions.

14. **Peer Support:**
   - Consider staying connected with hypertension support groups or communities. Sharing your experiences and learning from others can provide valuable insight and encouragement.

15. **Set New Goals:**
   - As you achieve your initial goals, consider setting new ones to continue improving your health and maintaining your victory over hypertension.

Long-term victory over high blood pressure is achievable with dedication and a proactive approach to health. By incorporating these strategies into your daily life and consistently monitoring and managing your hypertension, you can enjoy a healthier and more fulfilling future.

CHAPTER SIX
HEART-HEALTHY HABITS WITH HIGH BLOOD PRESSURE

Maintaining heart-healthy habits is crucial when you have high blood pressure (hypertension) or want to prevent it. These habits promote overall cardiovascular health and help control blood pressure. Here are some heart-healthy habits to consider:

1. **Follow a Heart-Healthy Diet:**
   - Embrace the Dietary Approaches to Stop Hypertension (DASH) diet, which emphasizes fruits, vegetables, whole grains, lean protein, and low-fat dairy products.
   - Limit your sodium (salt) intake to reduce the risk of high blood pressure and associated heart problems. Opt for fresh foods over processed ones, and use herbs and spices for flavor.
2. **Consume Adequate Potassium:**
   - Include potassium-rich foods in your diet, such as bananas, oranges, spinach, sweet potatoes, and beans. Potassium helps balance sodium levels and supports healthy blood pressure.
3. **Reduce Saturated and Trans Fats:**
   - Limit saturated and trans fats, which can contribute to high cholesterol levels and heart disease. Choose healthier fats, like those found in avocados, nuts, and olive oil.
4. **Fiber-Rich Foods:**
   - Increase your fiber intake by incorporating whole grains, fruits, vegetables, and legumes into your meals. Fiber can help lower blood pressure and improve heart health.
5. **Lean Protein Sources:**
   - Opt for lean protein sources, such as skinless poultry, fish, beans, and tofu. These choices are lower in saturated fats and better for heart health.
6. **Moderate Alcohol Consumption:**

- If you drink alcohol, do so in moderation. This typically means up to one drink per day for women and up to two drinks per day for men.

7. **Stay Hydrated:**
   - Drink plenty of water throughout the day to stay well-hydrated. Dehydration can affect blood pressure and overall health.

8. **Regular Exercise:**
   - Engage in regular physical activity, including both aerobic exercises and strength training. Aim for at least 150 minutes of moderate-intensity aerobic exercise or 75 minutes of vigorous-intensity aerobic exercise each week.

9. **Stress Management:**
   - Practice stress-reduction techniques like mindfulness meditation, deep breathing exercises, or yoga. Managing stress is important for heart health.

10. **Regular Monitoring:**
    - Monitor your blood pressure regularly, especially if you have hypertension. Keep a record of your readings and share them with your healthcare provider.

11. **Weight Management:**
    - Maintain a healthy weight or work on achieving and maintaining a healthy weight through a combination of diet and exercise.

12. **Adequate Sleep:**
    - Aim for 7-9 hours of quality sleep per night. Poor sleep can negatively impact blood pressure and overall heart health.

13. **Quit Smoking:**
    - If you smoke, seek support to quit. Smoking is a major risk factor for heart disease and high blood pressure.

14. **Limit Caffeine:**
    - If you're sensitive to caffeine, consider moderating your intake, as it can temporarily raise blood pressure.

15. **Regular Health Check-Ups:**
    - Attend routine check-ups with your healthcare provider to monitor your overall health and address any concerns.

16. **Medication Adherence:**

- If your healthcare provider prescribes medication, take it as directed and adhere to your medication schedule.

17. **Support System:**
    - Build a support system with family, friends, and healthcare professionals who can encourage and assist you in maintaining heart-healthy habits.

Adopting and maintaining these heart-healthy habits can go a long way in managing and preventing high blood pressure and reducing the risk of heart disease. Make these practices a part of your daily routine to support long-term cardiovascular health.

REGULAR HEALTH CHECK-UPS

Regular health check-ups are essential for individuals living with high blood pressure (hypertension). These check-ups help monitor your overall health, assess the effectiveness of your hypertension management plan, and detect any potential complications or risk factors. Here's a guide to regular health check-ups when living with high blood pressure:

1. **Frequency of Check-Ups:**
   - The frequency of check-ups may vary depending on the severity of your hypertension and your healthcare provider's recommendations. Generally, individuals with hypertension should have at least annual check-ups.
2. **Blood Pressure Monitoring:**
   - During each visit, your healthcare provider will measure your blood pressure. They will compare your readings to previous records to assess your blood pressure control.
3. **Medication Review:**
   - If you are taking medication to manage your blood pressure, your healthcare provider will review your prescription, its effectiveness, and any potential side effects. Be prepared to discuss any concerns or changes in your medication routine.
4. **Lifestyle Assessment:**

- Your healthcare provider will inquire about your diet, exercise routine, stress management practices, and any lifestyle changes you've made to manage your blood pressure.

5. **Physical Examination:**
   - A physical examination may be performed to assess your general health. Your provider will listen to your heart, check for signs of heart disease, and examine other relevant aspects of your health.

6. **Lab Tests:**
   - Blood tests may be ordered to check for cholesterol levels, blood glucose, and other metabolic markers. Elevated cholesterol and blood sugar levels can increase the risk of heart disease and impact hypertension.

7. **Kidney Function Assessment:**
   - Kidney function is often evaluated because hypertension can affect the kidneys. This assessment may involve measuring creatinine and glomerular filtration rate (GFR).

8. **Eye Examination:**
   - Regular eye exams can help detect eye problems related to hypertension, such as hypertensive retinopathy.

9. **Weight and BMI Measurement:**
   - Regularly monitoring your weight and calculating your Body Mass Index (BMI) is important for assessing weight management and overall health.

10. **Discussion of Symptoms:**
    - Share any symptoms or discomfort you've experienced, even if they seem unrelated to hypertension. These symptoms may provide clues to potential health issues.

11. **Review of Family History:**
    - Discuss any family history of heart disease, stroke, or hypertension with your healthcare provider. This information can help assess your risk and tailor your treatment plan.

12. **Stress Management:**
    - Talk about your stress levels and how you manage stress. Stress can impact blood pressure, so addressing it is important for overall health.

13. **Questions and Concerns:**
    - Use this opportunity to ask questions and express any concerns about your hypertension management or treatment plan.
14. **Vaccinations:**
    - Stay up to date with recommended vaccinations, including flu shots and vaccines that protect against pneumonia and other preventable diseases.
15. **Discussion of Lifestyle Modifications:**
    - Discuss any plans or challenges related to diet, exercise, smoking cessation, and alcohol consumption. Your healthcare provider can offer guidance and support.

Regular health check-ups provide an opportunity to address any issues or concerns promptly, monitor your progress, and make necessary adjustments to your hypertension management plan. Be an active participant in your healthcare, and maintain open and honest communication with your healthcare provider.

STAYING VIGILANT WHEN LIVING WITH HIGH BLOOD PRESSURE

Staying vigilant when living with high blood pressure (hypertension) is essential to effectively manage the condition and reduce the risk of complications. Here are some key strategies to help you remain vigilant in your hypertension management:

1. **Regular Monitoring:**
    - Continuously monitor your blood pressure as advised by your healthcare provider. Keeping a record of your readings helps you track your progress and detect any changes early.
2. **Adherence to Medication:**
    - Take your prescribed medication consistently and adhere to the schedule recommended by your healthcare provider. Skipping doses or discontinuing medication without

consulting your provider can lead to blood pressure fluctuations.

3. **Lifestyle Modifications:**
   - Maintain the heart-healthy lifestyle changes that have proven effective in controlling your blood pressure. This includes a balanced diet, regular exercise, stress management, and weight control.

4. **Dietary Awareness:**
   - Stay aware of your dietary choices and aim to limit sodium intake, consume potassium-rich foods, and maintain a diet low in saturated and trans fats.

5. **Regular Exercise:**
   - Keep up with your exercise routine, making it a consistent part of your lifestyle. Engage in both aerobic and strength training exercises as recommended.

6. **Stress Management:**
   - Practice stress-reduction techniques regularly to maintain a healthy response to stress. Mindfulness, meditation, and deep breathing exercises can be especially helpful.

7. **Weight Control:**
   - Maintain a healthy weight or work toward achieving and maintaining a healthy weight if needed. Being overweight can contribute to high blood pressure.

8. **Health Check-Ups:**
   - Attend routine health check-ups, and actively participate in discussions with your healthcare provider about your hypertension management.

9. **Medication Side Effects:**
   - Be aware of any potential side effects from your medication, and promptly report them to your healthcare provider. Your provider can adjust your medication or explore alternatives if necessary.

10. **Maintain a Support System:**
    - Continue to build and rely on your support system of family, friends, and healthcare professionals who understand and encourage your commitment to managing hypertension.

11. **Stay Informed:**

- Stay up to date on the latest developments in hypertension management and treatment, and be open to new strategies and recommendations.

12. **Regular Eye and Dental Exams:**
    - Schedule regular eye and dental check-ups. Eye exams can help detect hypertension-related issues like hypertensive retinopathy, while dental health is connected to overall well-being.

13. **Smoking Cessation:**
    - If you smoke, remain committed to quitting. Smoking is a major risk factor for heart disease and hypertension.

14. **Limit Alcohol:**
    - If you consume alcohol, do so in moderation. Excessive alcohol intake can raise blood pressure and have other adverse health effects.

15. **Healthy Sleep:**
    - Maintain healthy sleep patterns by getting adequate rest. Sleep is essential for overall well-being and blood pressure control.

16. **Emergency Preparedness:**
    - Be prepared for emergency situations by knowing how to respond if your blood pressure spikes. This may involve having a plan in place and knowing when to seek medical attention.

17. **Vaccinations:**
    - Stay current with recommended vaccinations, as they can help protect you from preventable diseases.

Staying vigilant in your hypertension management involves ongoing commitment to a heart-healthy lifestyle and consistent monitoring. It's essential to be proactive and informed about your health and to collaborate closely with your healthcare provider. By maintaining these vigilant practices, you can effectively control your blood pressure and reduce the risk of hypertension-related complications.

CHAPTER SEVEN
CONCLUSION

In conclusion, high blood pressure, or hypertension, is a common and serious medical condition that can lead to a range of health complications, including heart disease, stroke, and kidney problems. It's often referred to as the "silent killer" because it typically has no noticeable symptoms, making regular blood pressure monitoring and management critical.

Understanding high blood pressure is essential, and it's characterized by persistently elevated blood pressure levels. Blood pressure is measured with two values: systolic (the pressure in the arteries when the heart beats) and diastolic (the pressure in the arteries when the heart rests between beats). Ideal blood pressure is typically considered to be around 120/80 mm Hg.

There are two main types of hypertension:

1. Primary (essential) hypertension: This is the most common type, and its exact cause is often unknown. It is typically related to lifestyle factors and genetic predisposition.
2. Secondary hypertension: This type is usually caused by an underlying medical condition, such as kidney disease, hormonal disorders, or certain medications.

High blood pressure can have hidden dangers, as it's a major risk factor for cardiovascular diseases and other health problems. It's crucial to address and manage hypertension through a combination of lifestyle modifications and, in some cases, medication.

Effective management of high blood pressure involves:

- A heart-healthy diet that's low in salt and saturated fats
- Regular physical activity
- Stress management techniques

- Weight control
- Medications, when prescribed by a healthcare provider

Monitoring your progress, maintaining a support system, and staying vigilant in your hypertension management are also essential components of successful control.

In conclusion, with knowledge, commitment, and support, individuals living with high blood pressure can successfully manage the condition; reduce their risk of complications, and lead healthier, more fulfilling lives. Regular communication and collaboration with healthcare providers are key to achieving and maintaining healthy blood pressure levels.

ENCOURAGEMENT AND INSPIRATION TO PEOPLE LIVING WITH HIGH BLOOD PRESSURE

Living with high blood pressure (hypertension) can be challenging, but many people successfully manage their condition and lead healthy, fulfilling lives. Here's some encouragement and inspiration for those on this journey:

1. **You're Not Alone:**
   - Many people are dealing with hypertension, and there's a vast community of support and resources available to help you navigate this path. Reach out to others who understand your journey.
2. **Small Steps Lead to Big Changes:**
   - Every positive choice you make, whether it's eating a healthy meal, going for a walk, or managing stress, contributes to better blood pressure control. Small steps add up over time.
3. **Your Health Matters:**
   - Prioritizing your health is one of the most important decisions you can make. Your well-being affects not only you but also those who care about you.
4. **Progress Takes Time:**

- Managing hypertension is a journey, and it may require patience. Be kind to yourself, and remember that progress is not always linear.

5. **Celebrate Achievements:**
   - Celebrate your milestones, no matter how small. Whether it's a lower blood pressure reading or successfully sticking to your exercise routine, acknowledge your achievements.

6. **Stay Informed:**
   - Knowledge is power. Educate yourself about hypertension and its management. The more you know, the better equipped you are to make informed decisions.

7. **You Are Strong:**
   - Dealing with hypertension requires resilience and strength. You've already shown great courage by taking the steps to manage your health.

8. **Seek Support:**
   - Don't be afraid to reach out to your healthcare provider, family, and friends. You're not alone on this journey, and you can lean on your support system for encouragement and guidance.

9. **Adapt and Learn:**
   - Be open to adjusting your approach. If one strategy doesn't work, try another. Your journey is about continuous learning and adaptation.

10. **Advocate for Your Health:**
    - Be your own health advocate. Ask questions, share your concerns, and actively participate in your healthcare decisions.

11. **You're More Than Your Diagnosis:**
    - Remember that you are not defined by your condition. You have passions, interests, and dreams that make you unique. Continue to pursue your goals and live a full life.

12. **Visualize a Healthier Future:**
    - Imagine the positive impact your health improvements will have on your life. Visualization can be a powerful motivator.

13. **Support Others:**

- As you progress in your journey, you can inspire and support others who are facing similar challenges. Your experiences and insights can make a difference in someone else's life.

14. **Stay Vigilant, Stay Strong:**
    - Your commitment to managing hypertension is a testament to your strength and resilience. Continue to stay vigilant and persistent in your efforts.

Remember, you have the power to take control of your health and live a fulfilling life despite hypertension. Your journey is a testament to your determination and the choices you make every day to prioritize your well-being. Stay inspired, stay encouraged, and continue to work towards better health.

FUTURE RESEARCH DIRECTIONS ON HIGH BLOOD PRESSURE

Future research on high blood pressure (hypertension) is essential for improving our understanding of the condition and developing more effective strategies for prevention, diagnosis, and treatment. Here are some potential research directions in the field of hypertension:

1. **Genetic and Personalized Medicine:**
   - Investigate the genetic factors that contribute to hypertension and explore how personalized medicine can be used to tailor treatment plans based on an individual's genetic profile.
2. **Lifestyle and Behavioral Interventions:**
   - Research the most effective methods for promoting healthy lifestyle changes, such as diet, exercise, and stress management, to prevent and manage hypertension.
3. **Novel Blood Pressure Medications:**
   - Develop new classes of medications with fewer side effects and greater efficacy in controlling blood pressure. Research into innovative drug therapies is ongoing.
4. **Non-Invasive Blood Pressure Monitoring:**
   - Explore the development of non-invasive and wearable devices for continuous blood pressure monitoring, providing real-time data for individuals at risk of hypertension.
5. **Telemedicine and Remote Monitoring:**

- Investigate the use of telemedicine and remote monitoring tools to provide better access to healthcare and monitor blood pressure for individuals in remote or underserved areas.

6. **Early Detection and Screening:**
   - Develop and refine early detection methods and screening tools to identify individuals at high risk of developing hypertension.

7. **Hypertension in Vulnerable Populations:**
   - Research the unique challenges and risk factors for hypertension in vulnerable populations, such as low-income communities, racial and ethnic minorities, and individuals with limited access to healthcare.

8. **Hypertension and Mental Health:**
   - Examine the complex relationship between mental health and hypertension, including how stress, anxiety, and depression contribute to blood pressure levels.

9. **Precision Nutrition and Dietary Interventions:**
   - Investigate the role of precision nutrition and dietary interventions tailored to an individual's specific needs in preventing and managing hypertension.

10. **Management of Resistant Hypertension:**
    - Research into innovative approaches for managing resistant hypertension, which does not respond well to standard treatments.

11. **Hypertension and Pregnancy:**
    - Explore the impact of hypertension on maternal and fetal health, as well as ways to improve prenatal care and management.

12. **Patient Engagement and Education:**
    - Study the effectiveness of patient education and engagement programs in improving hypertension management and medication adherence.

13. **Hypertension and Technology:**
    - Investigate the use of digital health solutions, such as mobile apps and wearable devices, to support individuals in monitoring and managing their blood pressure.

14. **Environmental Factors:**

- Research the impact of environmental factors, including air quality, noise pollution, and climate change, on hypertension rates and outcomes.

15. **Global Health Initiatives:**
- Develop and implement global initiatives to address the growing burden of hypertension in low- and middle-income countries and underrepresented regions.

16. **Long-Term Cardiovascular Outcomes:**
- Study the long-term cardiovascular and renal outcomes in individuals who have successfully managed their hypertension to better understand the benefits of control.

Continued research in these areas will contribute to our understanding of hypertension, potentially lead to new and improved treatment options, and ultimately help reduce the global burden of high blood pressure and its associated health complications.

THE SIGNIFICANCE OF HIGH BLOOD PRESSURE AWARENESS

The significance of high blood pressure (hypertension) awareness cannot be overstated, as it has a profound impact on public health and individual well-being. Here are some key reasons why awareness of high blood pressure is crucial:

1. **Prevention and Early Detection:** Awareness is the first step in preventing hypertension and its associated complications. By educating the public about the risk factors and lifestyle choices that contribute to high blood pressure, individuals are more likely to make informed decisions to reduce their risk.

2. **Silent Nature of Hypertension:** Hypertension is often called the "silent killer" because it typically presents no noticeable symptoms. Without awareness and regular blood pressure monitoring, many people may not realize they have high blood pressure until it has already caused damage to their organs.

3. **Major Risk Factor for Cardiovascular Disease:** High blood pressure is one of the leading risk factors for heart disease, stroke, and other cardiovascular conditions. Raising awareness of its

significance can lead to better prevention and management of these life-threatening conditions.

4. **Global Health Burden:** Hypertension is a global health concern. Increasing awareness is essential for addressing this burden, particularly in low- and middle-income countries where it is on the rise.

5. **Cost-Effective Interventions:** Awareness campaigns can be highly cost-effective in preventing and managing hypertension. Promoting lifestyle changes and encouraging regular check-ups can reduce healthcare costs associated with treating hypertension-related complications.

6. **Empowerment:** Knowledge is empowering. When people are aware of their risk factors, the importance of regular blood pressure monitoring, and how to make heart-healthy lifestyle choices, they are better equipped to take control of their health.

7. **Reduced Complications:** Timely awareness and intervention can help prevent or delay hypertension-related complications, such as heart attacks, strokes, kidney disease, and vision problems.

8. **Quality of Life:** Controlling high blood pressure through awareness and management can significantly improve an individual's quality of life. This includes the ability to engage in physical activities, enjoy a fulfilling life, and reduce the need for multiple medications and medical interventions.

9. **Health Equity:** Raising awareness about hypertension is essential for addressing health disparities. Vulnerable and underserved populations often face higher rates of hypertension and related complications, and awareness campaigns can help bridge these gaps.

10. **Public Policy and Advocacy:** Hypertension awareness can drive public policy changes and initiatives aimed at promoting heart-healthy environments, access to healthcare, and interventions that support individuals in their journey to better health.

11. **Prevention of Hypertension-Related Mortality:** By raising awareness and encouraging individuals to seek medical care and lifestyle changes, hypertension-related deaths can be reduced.

12. **Fostering a Culture of Health:** Awareness campaigns help foster a culture of health in which individuals, families, and communities prioritize well-being and make healthy choices.

Conquering High Blood Pressure

In conclusion, the significance of high blood pressure awareness is paramount to public health, individual health, and the prevention of cardiovascular diseases. It empowers individuals to make informed decisions, seek early detection and intervention, and ultimately lead healthier, more fulfilling lives.